I
AM
PEACEFUL

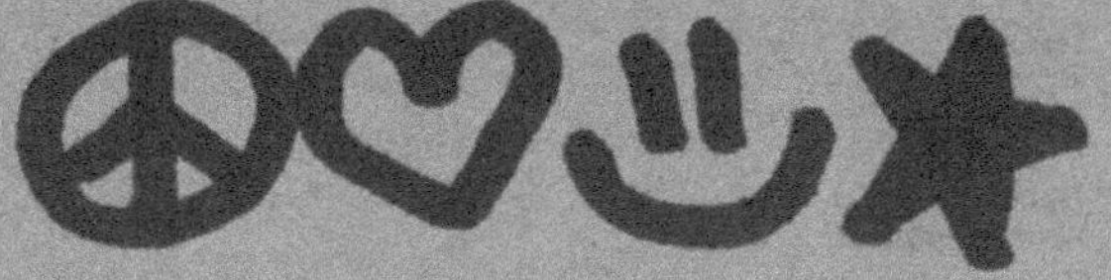

INTRODUCTION

Hello my beautiful, amazing, perfect friend! Yes! Perfect friend. 

I am grateful to be in this present moment with you. A moment of infinite possibilities and potential. A space of pure love and appreciation and total awareness of the miracle of life.

It has been more than five years since I first started following the original A to Z recipe. I committed each day to doing my best to check off all twenty-six exercises. It first started off with the intention of merely "checking" the proverbial box, before it turned into a hunger for fully understanding the importance of each and every letter.

When I first started the program, I was excited to experience a more enjoyable quality of life like the title suggested.

What I found after fully committing to the process was beyond words.

I found new levels of love, above and beyond my wildest dreams. This love is so much greater than any love I knew before, and there are no words in my limited vocabulary to describe them to you. You must fully experience this love yourself.

I discovered inner peace so deep that no matter what is going on in the world around me, I am able to stay grounded in the world within me.

I have cultivated happiness in such massive levels that rose-colored glasses and silver lining have turned into rose gold glasses and platinum lining.

I am experiencing levels of awareness that have taken my gratitude to the edge of the universe and back to the origin of space that exists in between the particles that make up each cell of my body.

I also became best friends with infinity. Yes, infinity and I are best friends. Through this friendship, I have been blessed with the wisdom that there is no beginning, and there is no end. There is only here and now. The intention of this life is to continue to grow, expand, and evolve in all directions mentally, physically, spiritually, and emotionally.

Within this book are the practices to experiencing a more enjoyable quality of life and taking this life to realms that have yet to be experienced.

As a reference point, allow me to provide some bullet points of what I found in this program:

First, when I started this program, I had yet to realize that I was excelling at some of the concepts, and I was severely deficient in other areas. That made some of these letters and exercises easy to master as part of my daily practice and created opportunities for vulnerability and surrender with other letters and exercises.

Some of my major breakthroughs occurred at ninety days of practicing the letter "X," which is forgiving a person, place, or thing. I then realized I needed to forgive myself. After another ninety days of forgiving myself, I experienced the freedom that comes with letting go of all of the baggage that I had been carrying around with me for years.

Another example is the letter "L", with the exercise of saying "I love myself" out loud 20x per day. After saying "I love myself" out loud twenty times a day, it finally became evident that I did—one year, four months, and twenty-eight days later. It took me about 10,260 repetitions. How do I know this was the day I fell in love with myself? Well, because this is the day where my thoughts, words, and actions were accepting and appreciative of myself—mentally, physically, spiritually, and emotionally. This granted me the awareness of my own perfection and allowed me to now see you in your perfection.

These are just two of the profound experiences that I have had since committing to this daily practice.

The best way I can explain the value of this practice is to compare it to golf. In golf, there are clubs, rules, courses, balls, earth, wind, fire, and water. The golfer then does the best they can with the tools they have to navigate the course with the intention of getting the ball in the hole with the least number of strokes.

To improve the golfer's odds, they can get the latest and greatest clubs. They can work with coaches. They can go to the driving range and practice their swing. They can go to the gym to increase their strength and mobility. They can study the game. They can go out and play. It appears through these principles that the golfers who fully commit to their practice are the ones who achieve at the highest level.

Every time they take the course, they face a new shot. Even if they are playing the same course that they have played many times. Each time they step up to the ball, there is a different position, a new hole placement, a variable wind, a temperature gradient, a different light, and at a subatomic level, the golfer is a different being mentally, physically, spiritually, and emotionally.

With all of these variables constantly shifting and changing, the golfer can only do the best they can with the tools they have at that moment in time. By practicing, they can increase their ability to succeed.

To me, this is true for life. Each year is a course, each day is a hole, and each breath is a stroke. Although I have experienced many Mondays, each one is unique, from the people I spend time with, the food I eat, the weather, the activities, and the placement of the sun, the moon, and the stars in the sky. The words, principles, and exercises in this book are the clubs I must practice with. Through this daily practice, I have learned to fully embrace the miracle that is life.

I invite you to do the same.

I have kept the letters the same as in this book as I did the first book, The Key to a More Enjoyable *Quality of Life From A to Z*. These letters are principles backed by science and theology. I have updated the meaning for each word based on the increased awareness that came from practicing the first book for so many years.

The biggest example of this is the letter "J: joke." The original book has the definition: "We all make mistakes; laugh at yourself, learn the lesson, and move on."

What I realized through the peace, love, happiness, and awareness that I have cultivated is there are no mistakes. A mistake is a judgment of an outcome that is different than what was desired. In a space free from judgment, I am able to look at each outcome and make an observation on my actions. I can then ask myself: Do I want a different outcome? If the Answer is yes, I must take different actions. If I am happy with the outcome, then I can continue taking the actions that are creating the experience.

"J: Joke" now reads: "I find joy every day in every way."

This change now puts my mind in a space of possibilities and opportunities to find joy in all of my interactions as I make my way through the day. Rather than focusing on one limited outcome and considering it a mistake, I am open to the awareness that it is just one outcome of infinite possibilities.

I have also gone through the book and updated the actions to help the development of new neural pathways. I added new books from experts in their fields; provided new songs that inspire the emotion of the word; and quoted someone who is highly recognized in embodying that particular concept.

Again, I would like to thank you for being on this life adventure with me. I know that all of the joy in my life only exists because of your existence in this universe with me. Each one of us creates ripples that allow the experience of life.

I look forward to the new peace, love, happiness, and awareness that will come from continuing this practice. May you and your family be blessed with

Peace

Love

Happiness

Infinite Abundance

—I am

A

ATTITUDE

I

CHOOSE MY ATTITUDE

ACTION: SMILE AND COUNT TO 20 BILLION

BOOK:
THE VICTORIOUS ATTITUDE
♥ ORISON SWEET MARDEI

SONG:
I GOTTA FEELING
♥ BLACK EYED PEASY

QUOTE:
ONE SMALL POSITIVE THOUGHT IN THE MORNING, CAN CHANGE YOUR WHOLE DAY.

♥ DALAI LAMA ♥

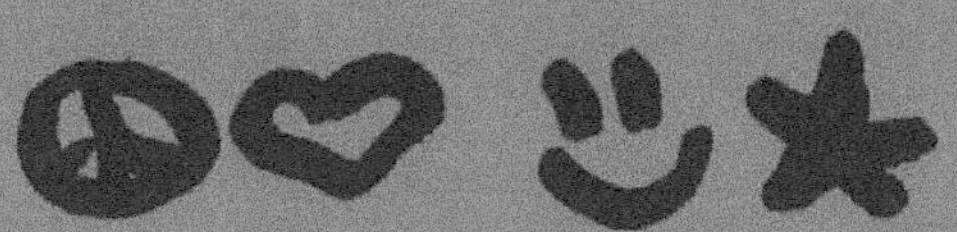

B

BREATH

I AM BREATHING

CONSCIOUSLY

ACTION: INHALE Love 10X EXHALE GRATITUDE

BOOK: ♥ THE SEVEN SPIRITUAL LAWS OF YOGA ♥ ♥ DEEPAK CHOPRA ♥

SONG: GRANDMOTHERSPHERE ♥ EAST FOREST ♥

QUOTE: REGULATE THE BREATHING, AND THEREBY CONTROL THE MIND. ♥ BKS IYENGAR ♥

C

CONFIDENCE
I AM
CONFIDENT

ACTION: SAY "I KNOW I CAN" 10X

BOOK: MIND GYM
✓GARY MACK✓

SONG: STANDING OUTSIDE THE FIRE
♥GARTH BROOKS♥

QUOTE: BELIEVE YOU CAN AND YOU'RE HALFWAY THERE
♥THEODORE ROOSEVELT♥

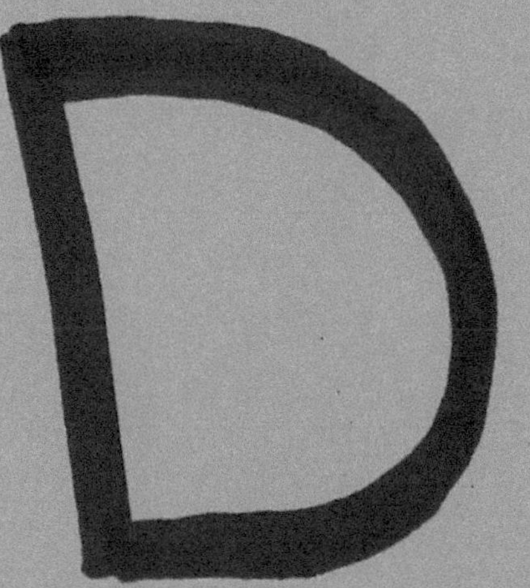

D

DETERMINATION
I AM
FOLLOWING
MY HEART

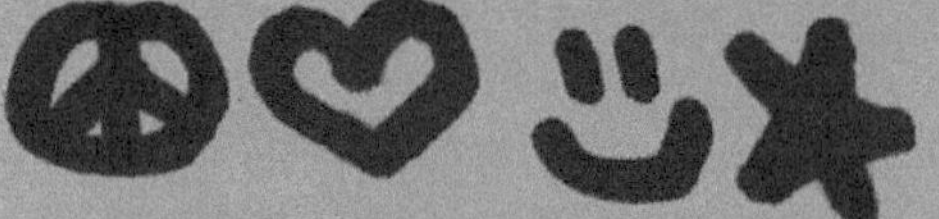

ACTION: SAY "I CAN I WILL" 10x

BOOK: RELENTLESS ♥Tim Grover♥

SONG: BELIEVER ♥IMAGINE DRAGONS♥

QUOTE: I BELIEVE SUCCESS IS ACHIEVED BY ORDINARY PEOPLE WITH EXTRAORDINARY DETERMINATION ♥ ZIG ZIGLAR ♥

E

EXERCISE

I MOVE
WITH
GRACE
AND
EASE

ACTION: +15 MINUTES OF MOVEMENT [SEE TRAINER JOE]

BOOK: BEYOND TRAINING ♥BEN GREENFIELD♥

SONG: JUMP ♥ VAN HALEN ♥

QUOTE: EXERCISE IS THE KEY NOT ONLY TO PHYSICAL HEALTH, BUT TO PEACE OF MIND. ♥NELSON MANDELA♥

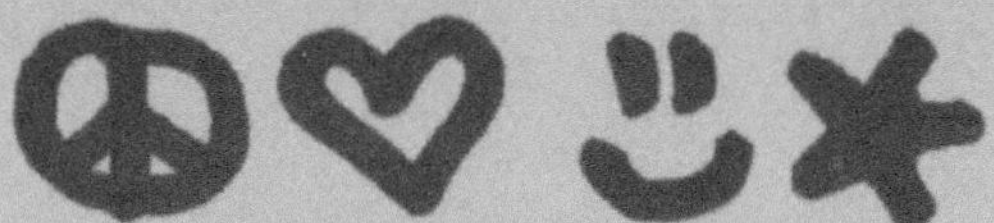

F

FAITH

FOLLOW
ALL
INTUITION
TO
HEAVEN

ACTION: PLACE BOTH HANDS ON YOUR ♡

BOOK: THE FREQUENCY
♥ LINDA WEST ♥

SONG: SOMETHING JUST LIKE THIS
♥ THE CHAINSMOKERS ♥
+
♥ COLD PLAY ♥

QUOTE: IT ALWAYS SEEMS IMPOSSIBLE, UNTIL IT IS DONE.
♥ NELSON MANDELA ♥

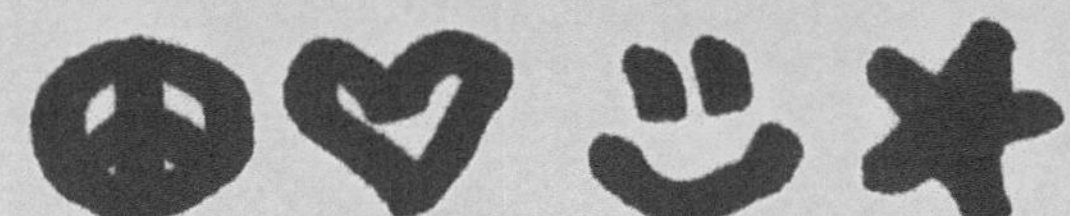

G

GRATITUDE
I AM
GRATEFUL
FOR WHERE
I AM

ACTION: SAY "THANK YOU" 20 X

BOOK: THE GO-GIVER
♥ BOB BURG + JOHN MANN ♥

SONG: GOOD LIFE
♥ ONE REPUBLIC ♥

QUOTE: ACKNOWLEDGING THE GOOD THAT YOU ALREADY HAVE IN YOUR LIFE IS THE FOUNDATION FOR ALL ABUNDANCE.
♥ ECKHART TOLLE ♥

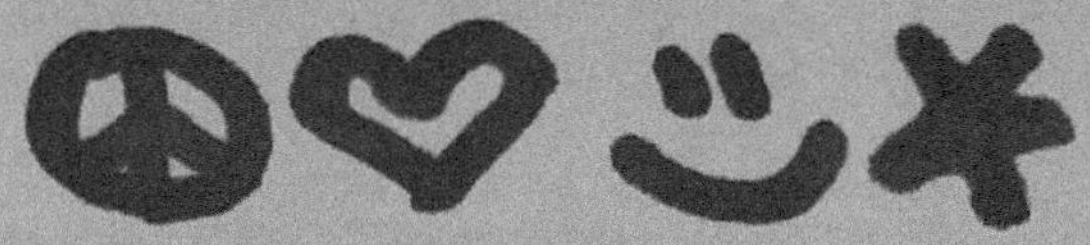

H

HELP OTHERS
I AM
HELPFUL

ACTION: PICK UP +1 PIECE OF TRASH / DAY

BOOK: ♥ START WITH WHY ♥ ♥ SIMON SINEK ♥

SONG: Love GENERATION ♥ BOB SINCLAR ♥

QUOTE:
HELP OTHERS ACHIEVE THEIR DREAMS AND YOU WILL ACHIEVE YOURS.
♥ LES BROWN ♥

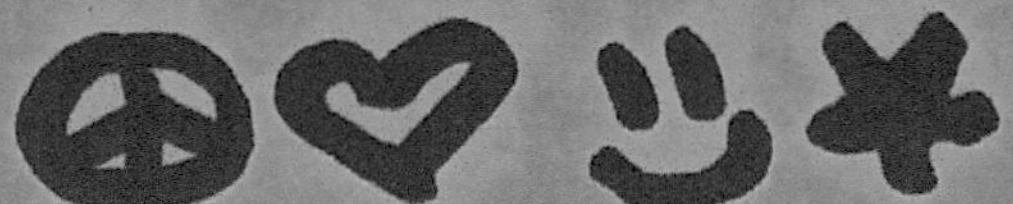

I

IMAGINATION

I

DREAM

BIG

ACTION: TAP YOUR 3RD EYE 10X

BOOK: THE MAGIC OF THINKING BIG
♥ DAVID SCHWARTZ ♥

SONG: ♥ A MILLION DREAMS ♥
ZIV ZAIFMAN & HUGH JACKMAN

QUOTE: LOGIC WILL GET YOU FROM A TO B. IMAGINATION WILL TAKE YOU EVERYWHERE.
♥ ALBERT EINSTEIN ♥

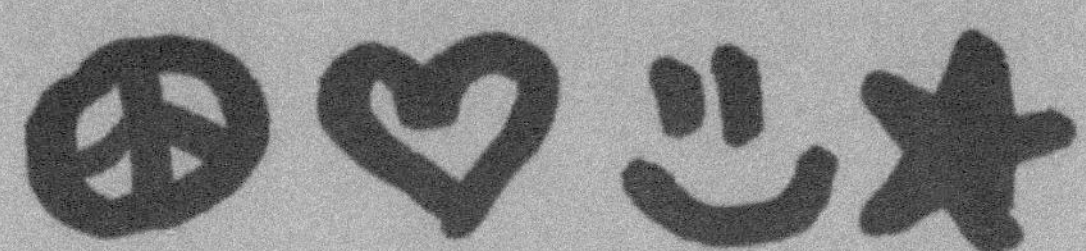

J
JOKE
I FIND JOY
EVERY DAY
IN
EVERY WAY

ACTION: SMILE AND TOUCH YOUR CHEEKS ☺

BOOK: DARING GRRTELY ♥BRENE BROWN♥

SONG: CELEBRATION ♥KOOL + THE GANG♥

QUOTE: LAUGHTER IS TIMELESS, IMAGINATION HAS NO AGE, AND DREAMS ARE FOREVER. ♥WALT DISNEY♥

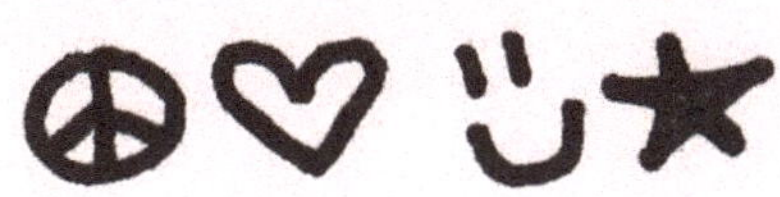

KINDNESS
I AM
KIND WITH MY
THOUGHTS, WORDS,
AND ACTIONS

ACTION: SAY A NICE THING ABOUT YOURSELF

BOOK: THE POWER OF MOMENTS ♥ CHIP + DAN HEATH ♥

SONG: YOU'VE GOT A FRIEND IN ME ♥ RANDY NEWMAN ♥

QUOTE: KINDNESS IS MY RELIGION. ♥ DALAI LAMA ♥

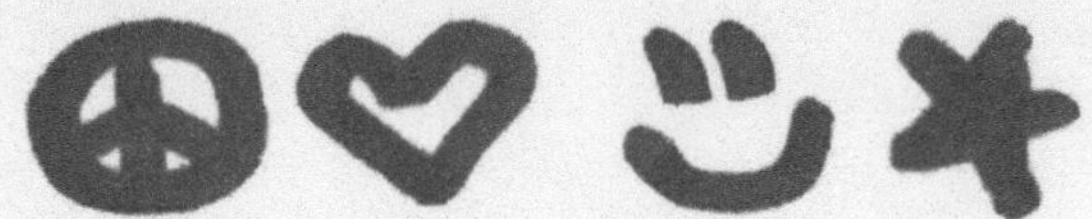

L
Love
I AM
Love WITH MY
THOUGHTS, WORDS,
AND ACTIONS

ACTION: TELL A FRIEND "I Love YOU"

BOOK: The Mastery of Love ♥Don Miguel Ruiz♥

SONG: IS THIS Love ♥Bob Marley♥

QUOTE: To fall in Love with Yourself is the first Secret to Happiness. ♥Robert Morely♥

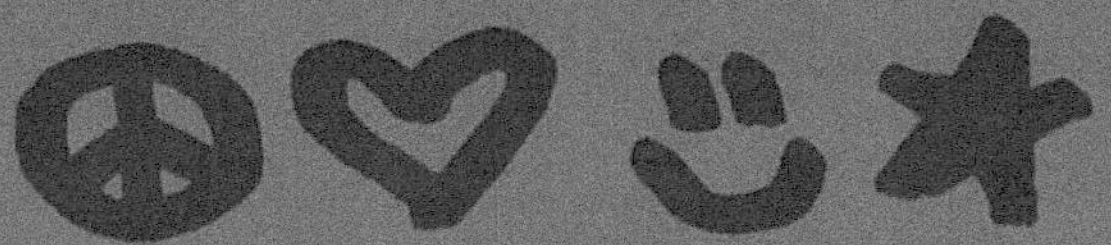

M

MANIFEST
I AM
AWARE OF MY
THOUGHTS

ACTION: TAP YOUR TEMPLES 10 X

BOOK: THE MASTER KEY SYSTEM ♥CHARLES HAANEL♥

SONG: LIFE IS WONDERFUL ♥JASON MRAZ♥

QUOTE: To MANIFEST YOUR HEARTS DESIRES YOU MUST BE WHAT YOUR HEART DESIRES ♥JOY PAGE♥

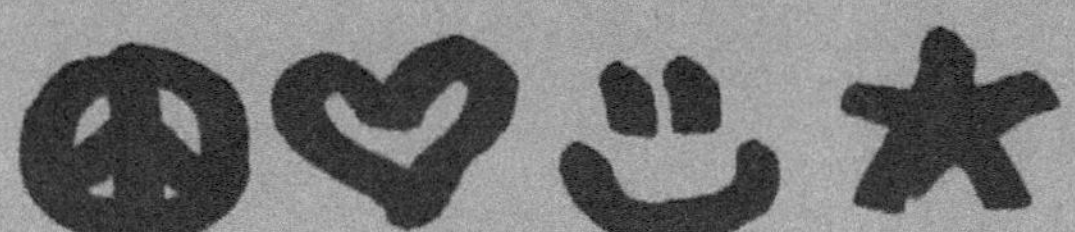

N

NUTRITION

I AM
WHAT I EAT,
I EAT FOR
SUCCESS

ACTION: FINISH EATING BY 8 PM

BOOK: Better Than Steroids ♥ Dr Warren Willey ♥

SONG: Good Foods ♥ Jack Hartmann ♥

QUOTE: The doctor of the future will no longer treat the human frame with drugs, but rather will cure and prevent disease with nutrition ♥ Thomas Edison ♥

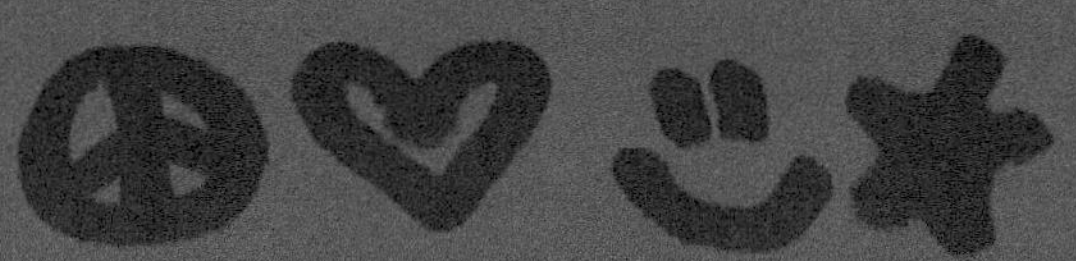

OPEN MINDED
I AM
AWARE EVERYONE
HAS THEIR OWN
REALITY + PERCEPTION

<u>**ACTION:**</u> OPEN YOUR EYES AS WIDE AS POSSIBLE

<u>**BOOK:**</u> SPARK ♥JOHN RATEY♥

<u>**SONG:**</u> WORLD HOLD ON ♥BOB SINCLAR♥

<u>**QUOTE:**</u> IF YOU WANT OTHERS TO BE HAPPY, PRACTICE COMPASSION. IF YOU WANT TO BE HAPPY, PRACTICE COMPASSION. ♥DALAI LAMA♥

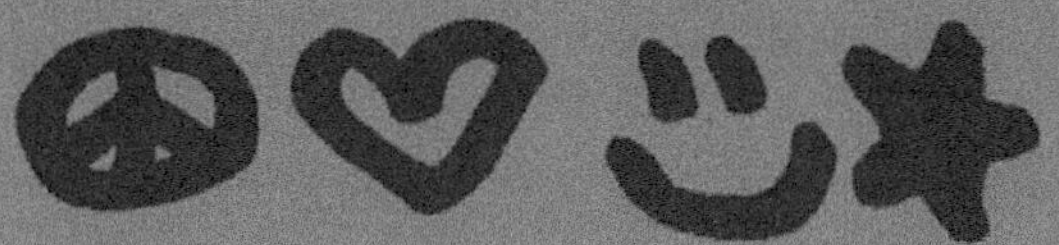

P

PURPOSE

I LIVE A LIFE FILLED WITH MEANING AND A STRONG PURPOSE.

ACTION: SAY YOUR PURPOSE IN THE MIRROR

BOOK: THE WAR OF ART ♥ STEVEN PRESSFIELD ♥

SONG: IF TODAY WAS YOUR LAST DAY ♥ NICKELBACK ♥

QUOTE: THE PURPOSE OF LIFE IS TO LIVE A LIFE OF PURPOSE. ♥ RICHARD LEIDER ♥

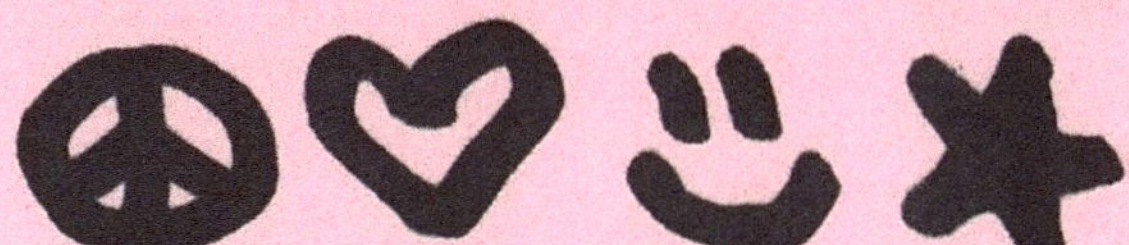

Q

QUIET TIME
I HAVE THE ABILITY
TO FIND PEACE +
STILLNESS WITHIN.

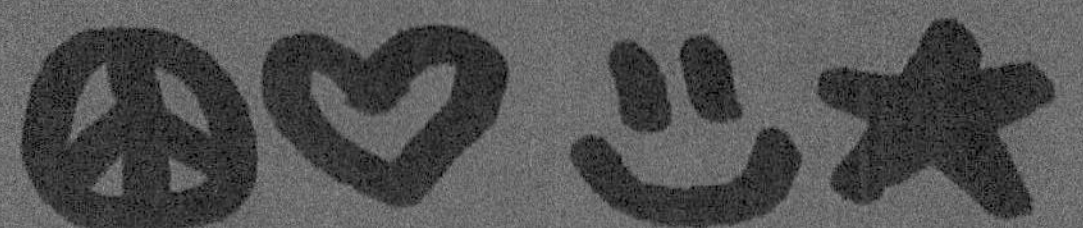

ACTION: +15 MIN OF STILLNESS

BOOK: STILLNESS SPEAKS ♥ ECKHART TOLLE ♥

SONG: A THOUSAND YEARS ♥ THE PIANO GUYS ♥

QUOTE: IN THE MIDST OF MOVEMENT AND CHAOS, KEEP STILLNESS INSIDE OF YOU.

♥ DEEPAK CHOPRA ♥

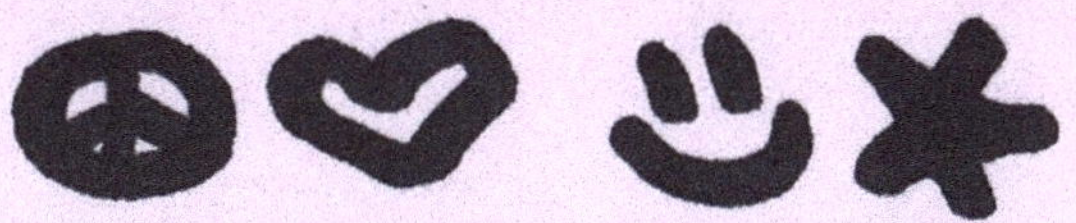

R

READ

READ KNOWLEDGE
THAT UP LIFTS AND
INSPIRES.

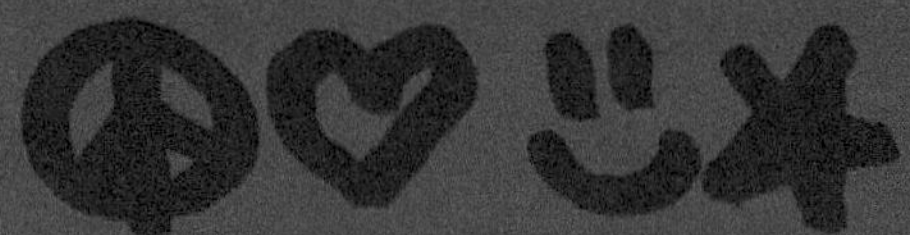

ACTION: +15 MINUTES OF READING DAILY

BOOK: SPIRITUAL WARRIOR ♥ JOHN ROGER DSS ♥

SONG: CLOSER TO THE HEART ♥ RUSH ♥

QUOTE: THE MORE THAT YOU READ, THE MORE THINGS YOU WILL KNOW. THE MORE THAT YOU LEARN, THE MORE PLACES YOU'LL GO. ♥ DR. SEUSS ♥

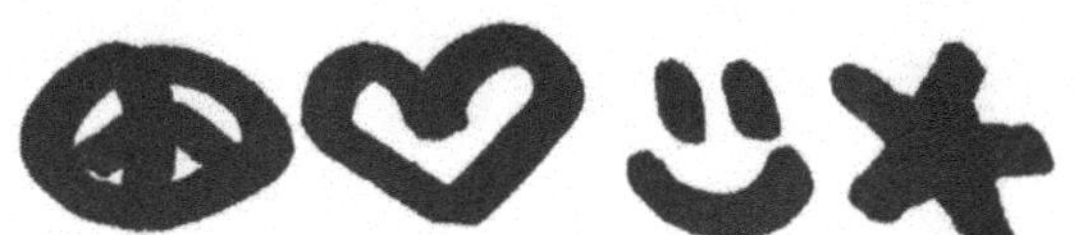

S

SLEEP

THE BODY ~~LOVES~~ TO RECHARGE, GET QUALITY CONSISTENT SLEEP.

ACTION: SAY 10 THINGS YOU ARE GRATEFUL FOR :)

BOOK: THE SLEEP REVOLUTION ♥ARIANNA HUFFINGTON♥

SONG: SILENT LUCIDITY ♥QUEENSRYCHE♥

QUOTE: BEFORE A DREAM IS REALIZED, THE SOUL OF THE WORLD TESTS EVERYTHING THAT WAS LEARNED ALONG THE WAY.

♥ PAULO COELHO ♥

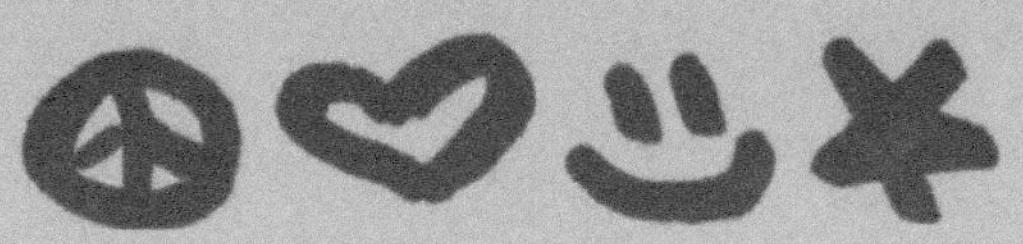

T

TOUCH
HEALS THE SOUL

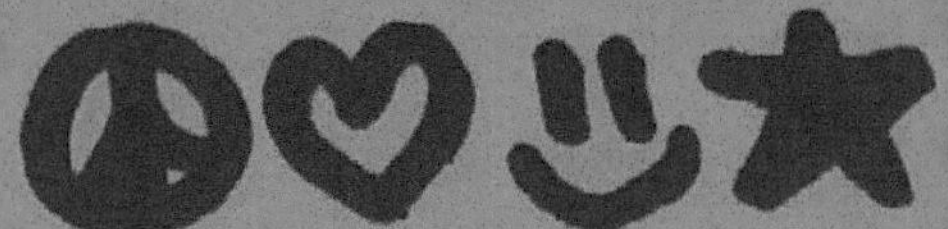

ACTION: MAKE EYE CONTACT FOR I MIN STRAIGHT

BOOK: THE TAPPING SOLUTION ♥NICK ORTNER♥

SONG: HOLD MY HAND ♥Hootie + The Blowfish♥

QUOTE: AT THE TOUCH OF ~~Love~~ EVERYONE BECOMES A POET. ♥PLATO♥

U
UNIQUE
I AM
THE ONLY ME
THERE EVER WILL
BE

ACTION: SAY "I AM" FROM Z → A

BOOK: FINDING YOUR OWN NORTH STAR ♥MARTHA BECK♥

SONG: ~~Love~~ MYSELF ♥HAILEE STEINFELD♥

QUOTE: I AM MORE MIRACULOUS THAN ANY COMBINATION OF WORDS, IN ANY LANGUAGE.
♥JOSEPH ROSEBERRY♥

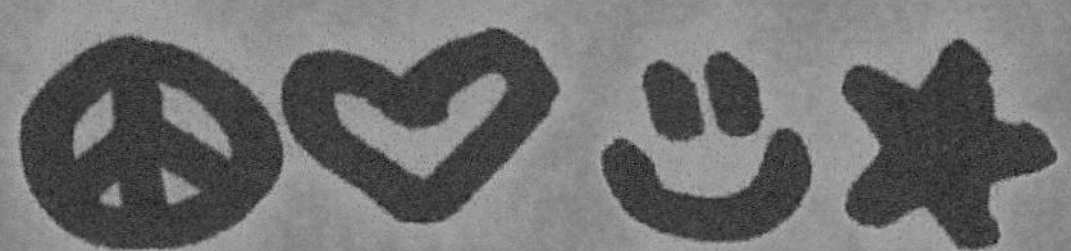

V

VISUALIZE

I SEE MYSELF
HAVING, DOING,
BEING MY HEARTS
GREATEST DESIRES

ACTION: CLOSE YOUR EYES + SAY "I AM SUCCESSFUL" 20X

BOOK: 'AS A MAN THINKETH' ♥ JAMES ALLEN ♥

SONG: FLASH DANCE WHAT A FEELING ♥ IRENE CARA ♥

QUOTE: PROPER VISUALIZATION BY THE EXERCISE OF CONCENTRATION AND WILLPOWER ENABLES US TO MATERIALIZE THOUGHTS, NOT ONLY AS DREAMS OR VISIONS IN THE MENTAL REALM, BUT ALSO AS EXPERIENCES IN THE MATERIAL REALM ♥ YOGANANDA ♥

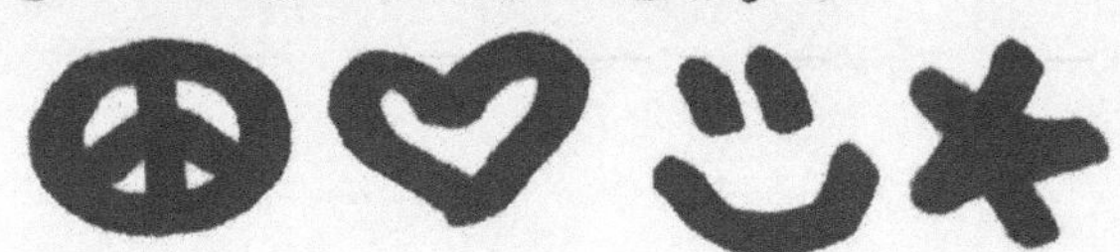

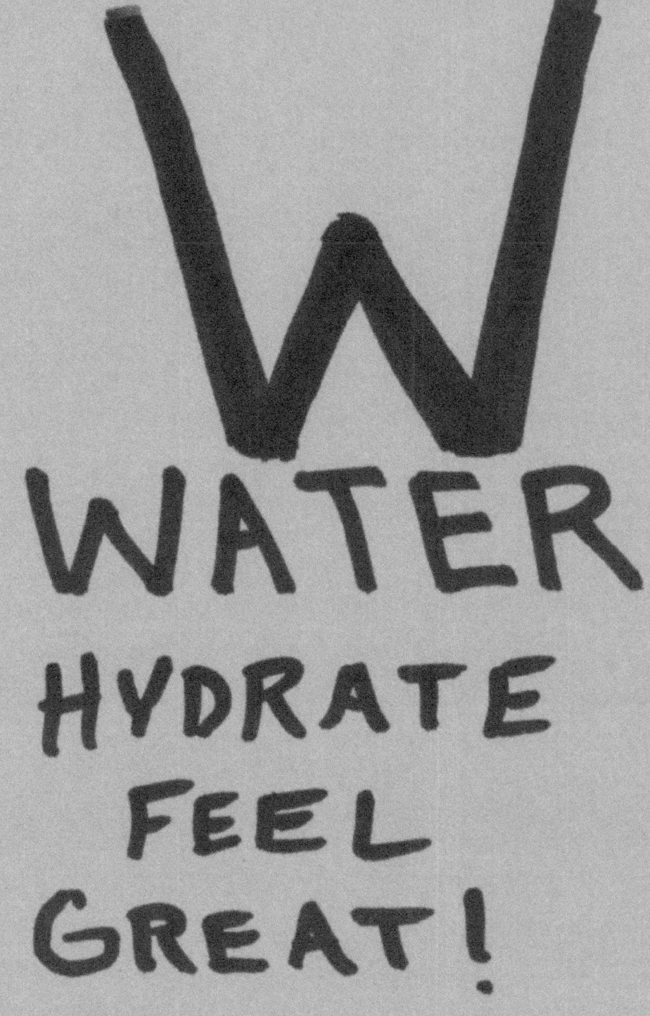
W
WATER
HYDRATE
FEEL
GREAT!
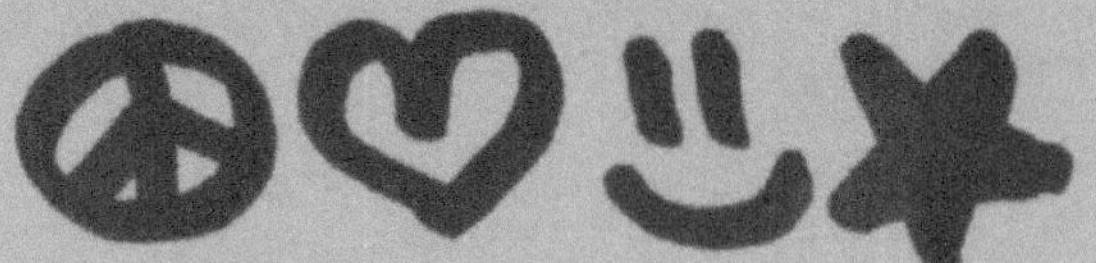

ACTION: SAY 'THANK YOU' BEFORE & AFTER EACH DRINK

BOOK: 10% HAPPIER ♥ DAN HARRIS ♥

SONG: THE HUMBLING RIVER ♥ PUSCIFER ♥

QUOTE: NOTHING IS SOFTER OR MORE FLEXIBLE THAN WATER, YET NOTHING CAN RESIST IT.

♥ LAO TZU ♥

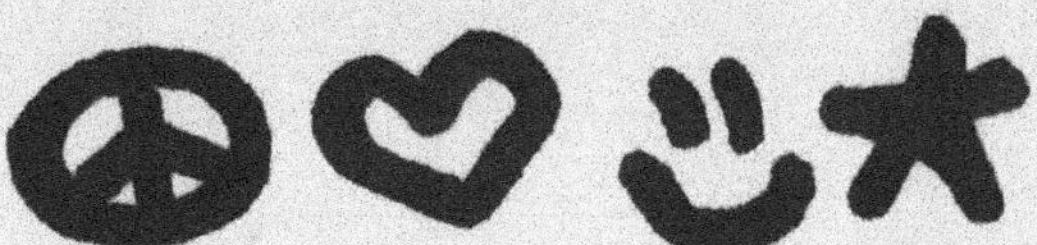

X-RAY VISION

I LOOK PAST THE SMOKE
I LOOK PAST THE MIRRORS
I SEE THE BEAUTY IN YOU
I SEE THE BEAUTY IN ME
I SEE THE BEAUTY IN
EVERYBODY!

ACTION: SEND A MESSAGE OF APPRECIATION TO A FRIEND :)

BOOK: THE POWER OF POSITIVE THINKING
♥ NORMAN VINCENT PEALE ♥

SONG: THANK U
♥ ALANIS MORISSETTE ♥

QUOTE: NO TWO LEAVES ARE ALIKE, AND YET THERE IS NO ANTAGONISM BETWEEN THEM OR BETWEEN THE BRANCHES ON WHICH THEY GROW.
♥ GANDHI ♥

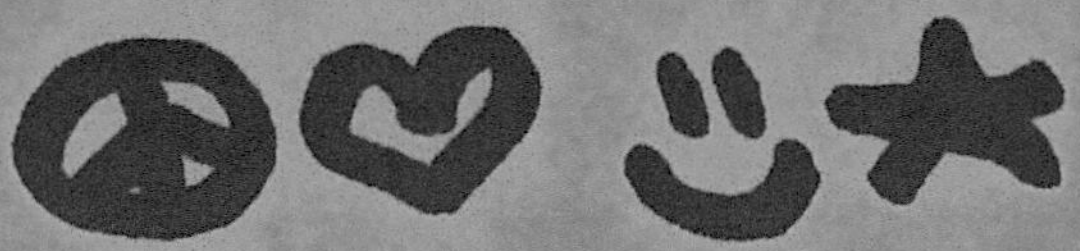

Y

YOGA

YOUR
ON
GOING
ADVENTURE

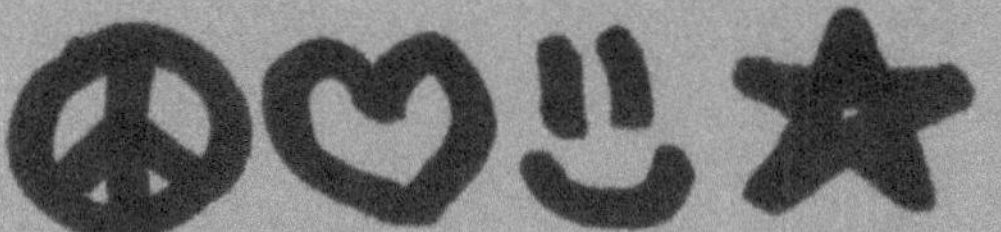

ACTION: +15 MINUTES OF STRETCHING PER DAY ☺

BOOK: THE SCIENCE OF YOGA ♥WILLIAM BROAD♥

SONG: I AM THE LIGHT OF MY SOUL ♥SIRGUN KAUR + SAT DARSHAN SINGH♥

QUOTE: MY SOUL HONORS YOUR SOUL. I HONOR THE LOVE, LIGHT, BEAUTY, TRUTH AND KINDNESS WITHIN YOU BECAUSE IT IS ALSO WITHIN ME. IN SHARING THESE THINGS THERE IS NO DISTANCE AND NO DIFFERENCE BETWEEN US. WE ARE THE SAME. WE ARE ONE. ♥NAMASTE♥

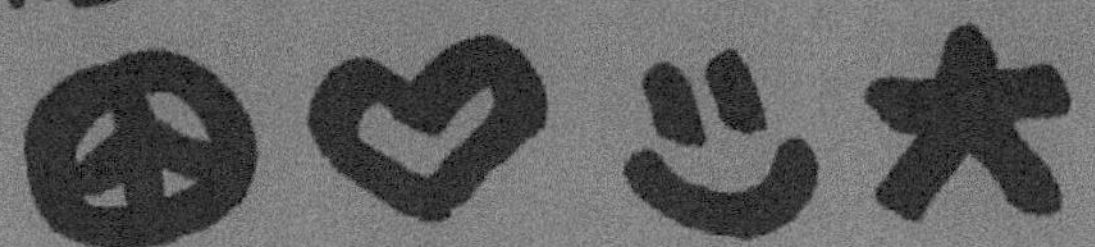

Z

ZEAL

THIS IS MY LIFE AND I CREATE IT WITH MY THOUGHTS, WORDS + ACTIONS.

<u>**ACTION:**</u> SMILE +TOUCH YOUR CHEEKS ☺

<u>**BOOK:**</u> A NEW EARTH ♥ECKHART TOLLE♥

<u>**SONG:**</u> THE GREATEST SHOW ♥HUGH JACKMAN♥

<u>**QUOTE:**</u> WELCOME TO YOUR LIFE!! ☺

♥ THE UNIVERSE ♥

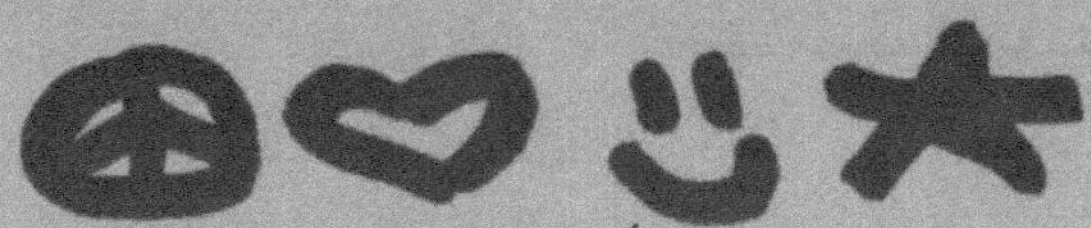

THE KEY TO INNER PEACE FROM A TO Z

A-Z	WORD	ACTION	CHECK
A	Attitude	Smile and Count to 20 Billion :)	
B	Breath	Inhale Love, Exhale Gratitude 10x :)	
C	Confidence	Say 'I Know, I Can!' 10x :)	
D	Determination	Say 'I Know, I Can!' 10x :)	
E	Exercise	15 Minutes of Movement per Day :)	
F	Faith	Place Both Hands on Your Heart :)	
G	Gratitude	Say 'Thank You' 20x :)	
H	Help Others	Pick Up +1 Piece of Trash/Day :)	
I	Imagination	Tap Your Third Eye 10x :)	
J	Joke	Smile and Touch Your Cheeks :)	
K	Kindness	Say a Nice Thing About Yourself:)	
L	Love	Tell a Friend 'I Love You' :)	
M	Manifest	Tap Your Temples 10x :)	
N	Nutrition	Finish Eating By 8pm :)	
O	Open-Minded	Open Your Eyes as Wide as Possible :)	
P	Purpose	Say Your Purpose in The Mirror :)	
Q	Quiet Time	15 Minutes of Stillness :)	
R	Read	15 Mintues of Reading :)	
S	Sleep	Say 10 Things You Are Grateful For Before Bed :)	
T	Touch	Make Eye Contact For 1 Minute Straight :)	
U	Unique	Say 'I Am' From Z to A :)	
V	Visualize	Close Your Eyes and Say 'I Am Successful' 20x :)	
W	Water	Say 'Thank You' Before and After Each Drink :)	
X	X-Ray Vision	Send a Message of Appreciation To a Friend :)	
Y	Yoga	15 Minutes of Stretching Per Day :)	
Z	Zeal	Smile and Touch Your Cheeks :)	

I
CHOOSE
PEACE